Table of Contents

I0425373

INTRODUCTION

Congratulations, you've decided to change your life. It might not seem like it now, but in less than 30 days you will feel like a brand-new person. This might seem intimidating, this might seem hard, this might even seem downright impossible. But when you trust your body and feed it the way that it needs to be fed, amazing things will start to happen.

So many people suffer. They suffer from sickness, depression, exhaustion, and excess weight. And sadly, going to the doctor generally means that you get medication not a solution. While sometimes medication is necessary to help our bodies, many times we have the ability to heal on our own. The only thing we lack is the knowledge to do so.

Inflammation is the underlying cause for many of today's top illnesses. Even though we might not realize it, a body that is riddled with inflammation is more prone to sickness, disease, and even death. The secret to stopping so many illnesses lies in stopping the inflammation. This is where the paleo diet comes in.

When you eat paleo, you are eating clean. You take everything processed out of your diet, no more sugars, nothing artificial, and most importantly nothing that your body can't naturally digest. In place of these unclean foods, you fill your body with organic fruits, vegetables, and high-protein meats. Even though this might sound like a bland diet, the good news is that many people have learned how to create delicious dishes from these simple foods and you can too.

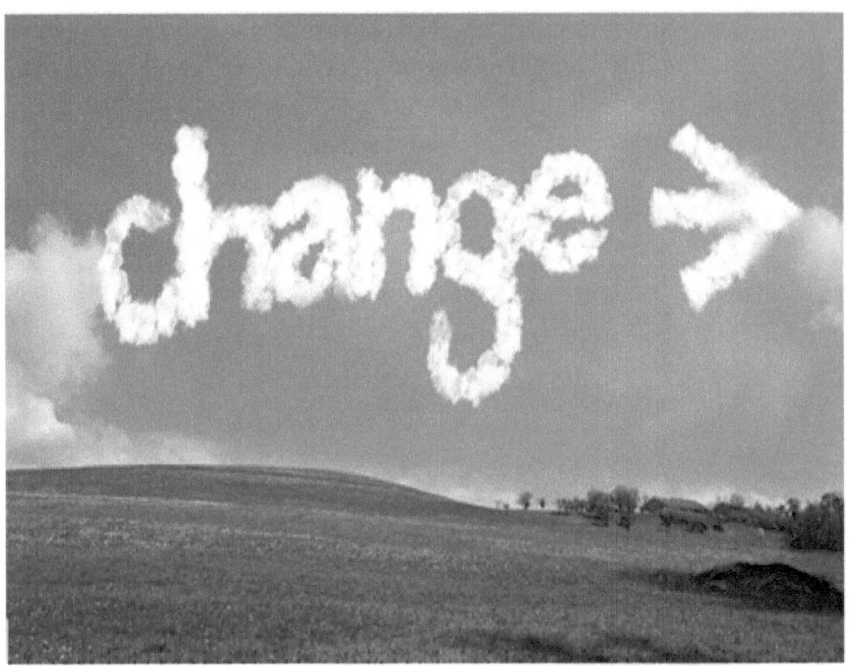

Because the paleo diet is so popular, you will be able to find people online and even in your community who are already on this eating path. And these people will be essential to your overall success. Reach out to them when you need to, ask questions, and remember everyone was once where you are now. The great thing about eating this way is that there is no shortage of support for you. Even if others in your home choose not to follow the paleo diet, you can still easily find the support you need.

One thing that is important to remember is that a transition will take time. Even though a month may not seem like that long, when you're just starting on this journey it can seem like an eternity. But if you have patience with yourself and you take the steps to transition slowly and gradually then success will be easier than you think. And once it becomes a habit, this way of eating will become part of your life. In fact, don't be surprised if you can't remember what your food journey was like before you started paleo.

Studies have shown that it takes 21 days to form a habit. If you can stick with this for 21 days you will develop a habit that will change your life. Less than a month from now the person in the mirror will be someone that you can only dream of today.

To Your Success!

What is the Paleo diet?

A Paleo diet, also known as a caveman diet dates back from about 2.5 million years ago and has been considered by many to vastly improve your health.

Following the paleo diet may lead to several health improvements which include, a healthy body composition, improved metabolic effects, lowers the rate of obesity and heart disease.

In a nutshell, you'll be eating what our ancestors ate thousands of years ago which is mostly whole foods as well as active lives. The diet has been proven to aid in weight loss.

You'll be exercising regularly while eating foods that are either hunted down or gathered. It is eating food in its most natural form just like humans did millions of years ago.

It helps you lose weight by stopping you from eating processed foods that have next to no minerals or vitamins and instead get you to change your diet to eating plenty of fruits and veggies.

By eating fruits and vegetables, you'll be giving your body a fighting chance to lose those unwanted pounds due to restricting certain food groups.

The paleo diet is not meant to be followed as a weight loss diet, but by eating healthy protein and fruits, you'll see a natural drop in weight.

When you think of Paleo, the general population would be thinking of eating nuts and seeds which is what gatherers ate, but it's advised to keep those to a minimum due to the high-calorie amount they contain.

How should you approach the Paleo Diet?

Millions of people around the world are obese, due to all the processed foods such as burgers, curries, pizza, desserts and alcoholic beverages that are easily available at local stores.

There are a wide variety of reasons why you may consider going Paleo, such as losing weight. But you need to remember that there is a right way to go paleo and a wrong way to go paleo. Here we will discuss the right way to go Paleo.

Right way – Avoid processed foods and eat real foods like vegetables, protein-based foods, and foods that contain healthy fats.

Wrong way – Make the change from fatty desserts to those considered healthy desserts as well as making your diet mostly fruits and potatoes.

The ultimate goal does not make any substitutes to your current diet by making the transition to fuel your body with clean whole foods.

Every time that you eat, you should be aiming at adding protein and a healthy amount of vegetables. You can eat fruit and sweet potatoes but eat them in moderation. By eating "paleo supplements," you're setting yourself up for failure.

Don't make an instant switch to real foods as this will cause you to burn and put the weight back on. It's recommended that you gradually make the change over two weeks as it allows your body to adapt to the way it handles all the new vitamins and minerals it's taking in.

CHAPTER 1

Your Mindset Matters

Have you ever wondered why some people have insane success and others don't? Sometimes two people can have the same education, the same background, and the same advantages and yet one person succeeds well above the other. Other times the person with all of the advantages has the hardest time finding success while the person with the least advantage is the one who takes everyone by surprise. How can that be?

The truth is there's one thing that sets success apart from failure, and it is not something that can be learned or something that can be taught. The truth behind the success of so many doesn't lie in their training, it lies in their mindset. And your food journey is no different.

If you go into your new eating journey with fear or intimidation, you're more likely to fail. If you go into this journey with doubt or feeling that you don't deserve this wonderful life you're trying to create for yourself, you're more likely to fail. But if you make the decision right now that paleo is the only way that you're going to eat for the rest of your life and there is no way that you ever could comprehend eating anything else, then you're setting yourself up for success

Talk to Yourself Kindly

Believe it or not, there is power in our thoughts. When we get frustrated with ourselves, when we get upset with ourselves, and we talk down to ourselves, all of that affects us on a subconscious level. Over time, the way you talk to yourself will change the way that you view yourself. Even if you simply make jokes at your expense, over time it can eat away at your self-esteem and sense of self.

Since you're starting this paleo journey, it's very important that you make the commitment to speak to yourself kindly from this point forward. Pay attention to the things that you say to yourself when you get frustrated, pay attention to your thoughts when you look in the mirror, and pay attention to the way that you allow others to treat you. You might be surprised at what you find out about yourself.

An easy way to practice being kind to yourself is to start every morning with some affirmations. This might sound silly, but after a couple of weeks of doing this, you will likely notice huge changes in the way you treat yourself. Use phrases like:

"My favorite feature is my..."
 "I love_____ about my body"
"I am proud of myself for..."
"I deserve to be healthy and happy"

Be Prepared for Bumps in the Road

Anytime you start a new journey there are going to be challenges, there's really no way around it. This doesn't mean you can't overcome them and it doesn't mean that they have to derail your journey. It simply means that you need to be prepared. Having a plan in place when times get tough is the best way for you to get through the rough patches easily.

For instance, if you've been eating a certain way your entire life you're asking a lot of your body, and your taste buds, to just start eating a new way. There are going to be times when you don't feel like doing this, there are going to be times when you have cravings, there'll even be times when you want to quit altogether. Believe it or not, a simple plan may be all you need to get through the rough stuff.

For example, one of the biggest pitfalls that many people face when trying to eat in a new way is letting themselves get hungry. After a hard day at work when you come home tired and starving, the last thing you want to do is go into the kitchen and prepare a meal... especially a meal you likely have never cooked before. But something as simple as having some pre-made snacks on hand can fill you up enough to get you through dinner prep.

Another major pitfall that many people experience when they're trying to change their eating habits is living with others who are eating differently. If you're the only one in your house that is eating clean it can be very tempting to fail when everyone around you is still eating the foods that you used to love. And this challenge can be even more difficult if you are the person who prepares the meals for your household. An easy way to plan for this obstacle is to batch prepare meals that can easily go into the freezer so that you can cook them quickly. This not only cuts down on your cooking time, but it will also make it much less tempting to eat what your family is eating if your meals can be ready at the same time.

Anytime that we let our bodies get hungry, it becomes so much easier to reach for what is close by. When things get tough, it's just easier to eat what is fast and familiar to us.

Making a plan for these obstacles now is going to help you to be successful in the future.

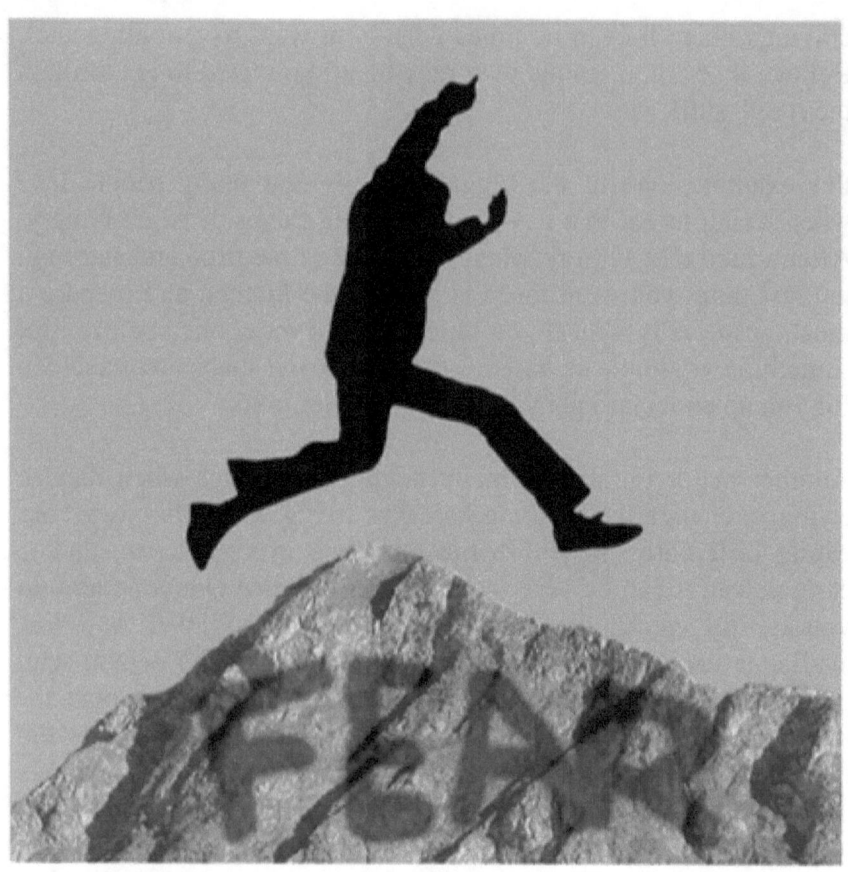

Create Your Goals

In addition to preparing for the bumps in the road, you also need to figure out what your goals are. As you go through your eating journey, your goals might start to change and that is okay. But if you don't have a starting point, a way to know where you began this journey, then you might not realize how far you've come.

While you are getting into the mindset of your new paleo journey, take some time to sit and think about what you want to accomplish. Are you looking to lose weight? Is there an illness that is currently affecting you? Are you looking for more energy? What things about yourself are you looking to improve by eating this way?

Your answers are your own, they are personal to you and you alone. But defining these goals before you go any further will help you in the long run. It's a good idea to take some time now and make a list of everything you want to accomplish. It's also a good idea to check in with your goals at least once a week to make sure you stay on track.

If your goals change, remember that's okay too, it just means you're progressing in your journey :)

CHAPTER 2

Starting Steps

So now that you have your mind set in order, it's time to start concentrating on something more fun. This is the part of your journey where you're going to go through your home and get everything ready for your paleo success. And where things get exciting! Once you're done with your starting steps, you have everything you need set in place for your lasting success.

Create Your Meal Plan

The first thing you need to do is create your meal plan. The reason it's important to do this first is that your meal plan will let you know what food you need to have in the house, what you need to shop for, and what snacks you can prepare in case of an emergency.

Since most people live on a budget, it's often easier to make a meal plan for the length of time between your paychecks. Since you'll be eating many fruits and vegetables, you will likely go to store more than once before your next paycheck, but having a budget to work with will ensure that you don't run out of paleo meals without a way to replace them.

So let's say there are two weeks between now and your next pay cycle, you will make a two-week meal plan. Each day of the plan you will allow yourself breakfast, lunch, dinner, and snacks. In the beginning, it's best to stick with ingredients that you're familiar with, and meals that are easier to prepare. But as you get more comfortable, you will fall into your own meal routine and it will not take you nearly as much time to create your meal plan each week.

Your Kitchen Clean Out

Once you know what you're going to be preparing, it's time to start cleaning out your kitchen. The reason it's best to wait until you have a meal plan to start cleaning the kitchen out is that you want to be sure that nothing you need accidentally gets thrown away.

Obviously, when you clean out your kitchen, you want to get rid of anything processed and any junk food. But it doesn't stop there, you will have to go through your freezer and refrigerator and start looking at food labels. You might be surprised to find that even some "healthy" foods contain ingredients that are actually unhealthy. Rather than throwing these foods out, it may be a good idea to save them for a local food pantry.

Once you have your newly cleaned out kitchen, it might be very tempting to go out and start buying healthy food items to fill it up. As tempting as that is, you want to hold off just a little bit longer. Sometimes we buy things, even healthy things, that we don't already have a plan to use. Many times this leads to the food going bad. Even though your fridge might look a little bit bare for the first few weeks of your paleo journey, as long as you have the food to create the meals and the snacks that you need it's best to resist the temptation to buy more.

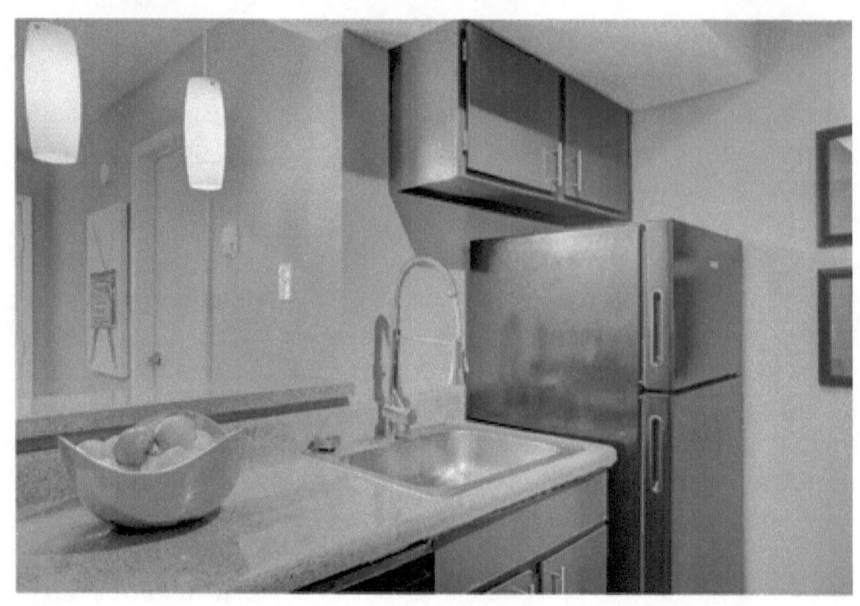

Make Your Shopping List

Once you've cleaned out your kitchen, it's time to focus on making your shopping list. While your first trip to the store might seem overwhelming, over time your new shopping habits will become natural.If there are any items on your shopping list that you are unfamiliar with, it might be a good idea to Google them now while you're at home. A simple Google search can help you figure out what the ingredient is used for and even where to find it in the store.

Additionally, if there are both paleo and non-paleo versions of this ingredient, a bit of Google research can help you find the paleo brand that you should be using.

Since you will likely begin making certain meals a staple in your new diet, it might be a good idea to organize your shopping list. For example, an Excel spreadsheet will help you to break down all of your items by the section of the store they belong to, and this will allow you to get through the store more quickly.

CHAPTER 3

Paleo Foods

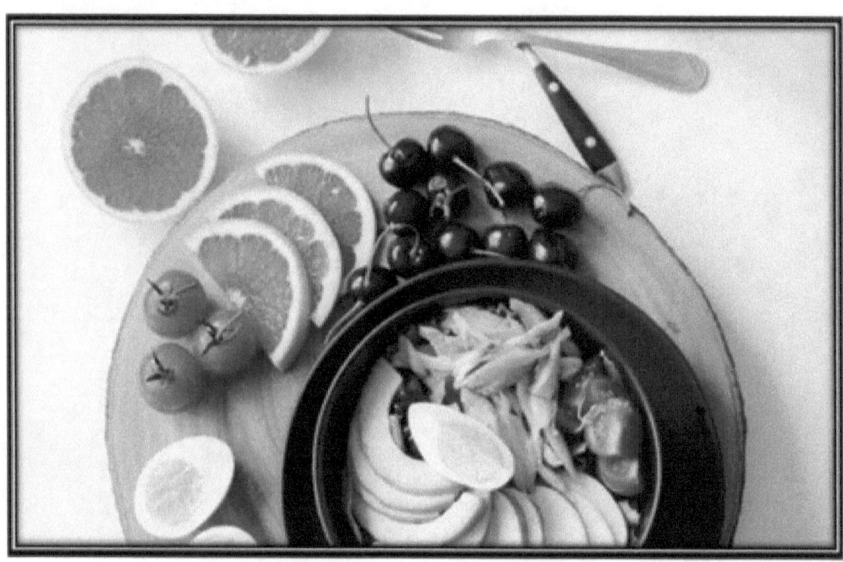

The general rule is to have organic, unrefined, and grass-fed or pasture raised foods. You're allowed as much real, unprocessed foods as possible. With a wide range of recipe ideas, you have access to an extensive range of delicious, fulling yet wholesome, healthy good food.

Allowed Foods

Below is a list of foods that will help you get on the right track to living and eating the Paleo lifestyle.

Meats: Eat beef, chicken, lamb, pork, etc.

Vegetables: You can consume fresh green vegetables such as kale, spinach as well as cauliflower, broccoli, peppers, onions, tomatoes, and carrots.

These are rich in vitamins, minerals, antioxidants, and phytonutrients. They reduce the several degenerative diseases developing such as diabetes, neurological decline, and cancer.

Fruits: Fresh, ripe, tasty and colorful fruits such as apples, oranges, bananas, pears, strawberries, blueberries, pineapples and more, are bonuses to the diet as no matter what your preference might be, you would undeniably find your choice among the list of fruits available.

Fish and Seafood: Have wild-caught fish such as salmon, shrimp, trout, shellfish, etc.

Eggs: Always make Omega-3 enriched eggs part of your diet. Several studies have proved that diets rich in Omega-3 fats reduce, in a significant way, cancer, obesity, heart disease, cognitive decline, diabetes, etc.

Healthy Fats and Oils: You can also add oils like coconut oil, olive oil and avocado oil to your diet.

Salt: Only consume sea salt or Himalayan salt.

Water: Water is an essential component of a balanced diet. Ensure you drink plenty of water and make sure that you always stay hydrated.

Tea and Coffee: It is okay to have tea and coffee as they are rich in antioxidants. Green tea is considered to be particularly healthy. Tubers: Eat potatoes in moderation, yams, turnips, and sweet potatoes.

Nuts and Seeds: Almonds, hazelnuts, walnuts, pumpkin seeds but in moderation as they contain many calories. One of the benefits of nuts is that they fill you up and leave you feeling fuller for longer.

Dark Chocolate: Dark chocolate with high cocoa content is considered to be very nutritious as well as tasty. It's a delicious indulgence to have.

Foods You Should Avoid

You can't eat processed foods on this diet. And since our ancestors were hunter- gatherers, not farmers, say goodbye to wheat and dairy, along with other grains and legumes (such as peanuts and beans).

Foods that contain the following ingredients should be avoided as well as the following:

Dairy: Avoid milk and dairy products completely. However, some Paleo recipes include butter and cheese, which are full-fat diaries. Artificial Sweeteners: Sucralose, Saccharin, and potassium. Natural sweeteners can be used instead.

Grains: Wheat, bread and pasta, as well as rye, barley should be avoided at all cost.

Legumes: Beans, and lentils

Vegetable Oils: Sunflower oil, soybean oil, cottonseed oil, grapeseed oil, and safflower oil.

Trans Fats: Also known as partially hydrogenated oils, they're found in various types of processed foods of which margarine is a good example.

CHAPTER 4

Your Week One Plan

Congratulations, you have officially started your paleo journey. After reading the previous chapters, you have everything set in place to give you a successful start to this new eating path. It might be very tempting to dive in headfirst right now, after all, you've set up your house, you set up your life and gotten rid of anything that does not adhere to your new way of eating. Believe it or not, the worst thing you can do right now is completely change your way of eating all at once. This will set you up for failure. Instead of going "all in" this week, you are urged to begin your transition slowly.

Start Small

The easiest way to develop a new habit is to take it piece by piece. This way you can allow your body and mind to adjust and adapt to the changes you are making in your life. Once the first piece becomes a natural habit in your daily life, it's time to add on a second piece. As that second piece becomes a natural habit, you will layer on a third piece. And so you will keep going until this way of eating becomes your new way of life.

So what does starting small mean? It can mean different things to different people. For instance, if you're very physically active and you are already eating very clean, then starting small might be eating full paleo three days out of your week.

On the other hand, if you're brand-new to eating clean then your body and mind might be overwhelmed if you make the commitment to eat fully paleo three days a week. The reason is that you may be adjusting to a completely new way of eating. Instead of minor changes to your diet, you will likely be retraining your taste buds altogether. Starting small for you might be something as simple as eating one paleo snack each day.

Focus on Your Breakfast and Morning Drinks

For most of us, we are right in the middle of eating completely unclean foods and eating completely clean foods. Because of this, if you're unsure what starting small means to you then it is a good idea to start taking your day one chunk at a time.

During week one, focus on nothing but breakfast and your morning drinks. The thought of making paleo breakfasts might seem intimidating right now, but just one or two simple breakfasts can get you through the week. Most likely, these simple breakfasts will also be come a staple meal for you.

A good baseline for your paleo breakfast is eggs. These can be combined with sweet potatoes, hard-boiled, or used to make a filling frittata. In fact, eggs are a staple in the paleo diet and it's not a bad idea to always keep extras on hand.

Start Getting Comfortable in Your Kitchen

For many of us, the thought of preparing meals in the kitchen can be a bit overwhelming. Between work and kids and the general craziness of life, most of us know how to heat up food or prepare quick meals but we are at a loss when it comes to making clean and healthy meals that require a bit of preparation.

The good news is even if you've never been comfortable in your kitchen, it's still not too late to start. Begin by finding simple recipes that you're familiar with and comfortable making, and then take a day or two out of each week to try your hand at more complicated recipes that interest you.

CHAPTER 5

Your Week Two Plan

If you made it to week two, the good news is that you're well underway to your new lifestyle. Week one might have been awkward. It may have been a bit time-consuming, and it might've taken more preparation than you wanted, but the good news is you've laid the foundation and all you have to do is follow it.

One of the good things about transitioning slowly is that it allows your body to detox slowly. In other words, you will likely be spared many of the detox discomforts that come when you throw your body into a cleansing state too quickly. However, you might still find that you are feeling some mild detox symptoms. Things like headaches, stomach upset, and fatigue can all be signs that your body is in a detox state. This shouldn't last long, and once you get through it you will likely feel better than you have in years.

Your Week Two Focus

Now that it's week two, it is time to add a second layer to habits that you are building. This week you will continue to focus on your morning drinks and your breakfasts. Just like last week, these meals should be paleo friendly, and rather than looking for new recipes, it may not be a bad idea to duplicate the breakfasts and morning drinks that you had last week.

This week you will add lunch to the mix. So, you will spend the majority of your day eating and drinking clean. Paleo lunches don't have to be hard and 'can be as easy and simple as a cobb salad with a paleo friendly dressing. Things like hard-boiled eggs, bacon, and avocados help you feel full for that long stretch between lunch and dinner.

It might not be a bad idea to just stick with salads for the entire week. Choosing three types of salad and prepping them beforehand will give you quick go-to meals without keeping you chained to your kitchen.

Cheating Urges

It's not uncommon at this point in the game to be missing the foods that you used to eat. This is where things can get tricky, and where many people will start to slip in their new way of eating. But with a few simple tricks, you can get through these bumps with ease.

For instance, as we discussed before having pre-made meals on hand is essential. This will prevent you from reaching for the closest food out of hunger. It may not be a bad idea to do some research on paleo snacks and try your hand at creating some. Additionally, anything that can be frozen will last longer while still being accessible to you when you need it.

If you absolutely must cheat, it's best to wait until dinner. This way the clean foods that you ate for breakfast and lunch will have already had a chance to work through your system and won't get clogged up by the unclean foods that are likely slow moving in the digestive tract.

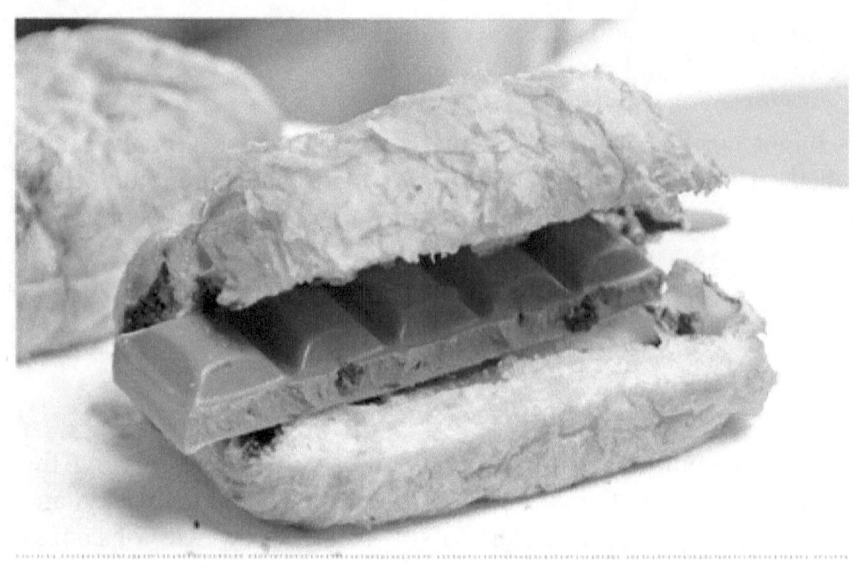

CHAPTER 6

Week Three and Beyond

The great news is if you made it to week three then all of this is becoming child's play. In other words, many of these new eating routines are becoming a habit. Because of this, in many ways, your last week will be the easiest week. This is where we will layer the last piece of your new healthy eating foundation.

As you've probably guessed, during this week we are going to focus on eating all meals paleo. If you're stumped at what to make for dinner, consider making something that you've already become comfortable with during weeks one and two. For instance, a simple breakfast dinner or hearty dinner salad will be easy to fix and you most likely already have the ingredients on hand.

If you still feel like there are times when you may be eating non-paleo, do your best to schedule those meals. Meaning, if you know you will be out of town or at a wedding then you know the chances are good that you will have to pre-make your meals or go off paleo during that time. It's a great idea to prepare for these things beforehand by making your own paleo friendly snacks and meals that can be eaten cold. And as discussed, if you're still not able to avoid eating non-paleo, try to eat that unclean meal at dinner.

Positive Effects

By now, you're very likely feeling the positive effects of the changes you've been making. Don't be surprised if you find yourself with more energy, better concentration, and even clearer skin. Because you've been eating this way, you have allowed your body to rid itself of old waste. And because of this, your body's energy can now be used to keep you healthy from this point forward.

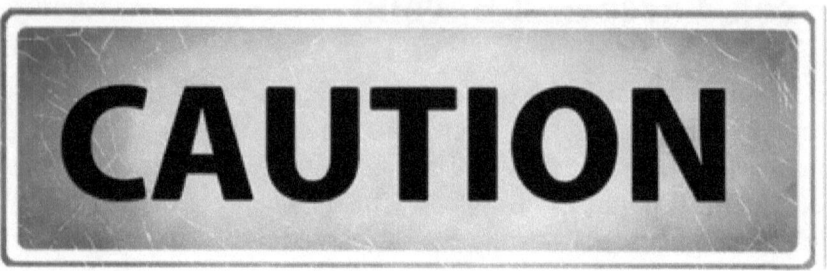

A Word of Caution

One thing you might want to be aware of is that anytime you eat unclean your body will likely let you know. Even foods that you once loved might now cause you to be sick. In fact, foods that you once loved may even taste very different than you remember them.

Because your body has already gone through a detox process, it has basically been reset. While all this is a good thing, it can also cause frustration if you are not prepared for it.

One option that many paleo eaters opt to do is find paleo versions of the old foods that they loved. This takes a bit of creativity, but there are many places online that will give you tips, recipes, and inspiration. In fact, paleo is so popular that pretty much everything has a paleo alternative.

Things like macaroni and cheese, rice, and even doughnuts can be paleo friendly with a few simple tweaks. And in many cases, a simple ingredient swap is all that you need to turn your favorite meals paleo.

Weekly Diet Plan

To help you ease into the Paleo diet, below is a quick plan you can use. This is just an overall plan and will need adjusting based on your current build and dietary preferences.

Monday

• Breakfast: Eggs and vegetables lightly sauted with coconut oil (MCT oil)
• Lunch: Chicken salad with olive oil and a small portion of nuts
• Dinner: Burgers (steamed) with vegetables, but exclude the bun.

Tuesday

• Breakfast: Bacon and eggs, with a small portion of fruit.
• Lunch: Leftover burgers from Monday.
• Dinner: Butter fried salmon and a side portion of vegetables.

Wednesday

• Breakfast: Leftover meat with vegetables.
• Lunch: Meat sandwich wrapped in lettuce.
• Dinner: Beef and vegetable stir-fry.

Thursday

• Breakfast: Eggs and a piece of fruit.
• Lunch: Leftover stir-fry from the night before. A handful of nuts.
• Dinner: Fried pork with vegetables.

Friday

- Breakfast: Eggs and vegetables sauted in coconut oil.
- Lunch: Chicken salad sprinkled with crush almonds.
- Dinner: Steak with vegetables and sweet potatoes.

Saturday

- Breakfast: Bacon and eggs with a piece of fruit.

- Lunch: Leftover steak and vegetables from the night before.

- Dinner: Baked salmon with vegetables and slices avocado.

Sunday

- Breakfast: Leftover meat with vegetables.
- Lunch: Meat sandwich wrapped in lettuce.
- Dinner: Beef and vegetable stir-fry.

Ultimately what you need to remember is that you need to think like hunter-gatherers, eating foods that they would've eaten. Remember there was no Pizzahut or McDonald's millions of years ago, so avoid processed foods at all costs.

CHAPTER 7

Exercise and The Paleo Diet

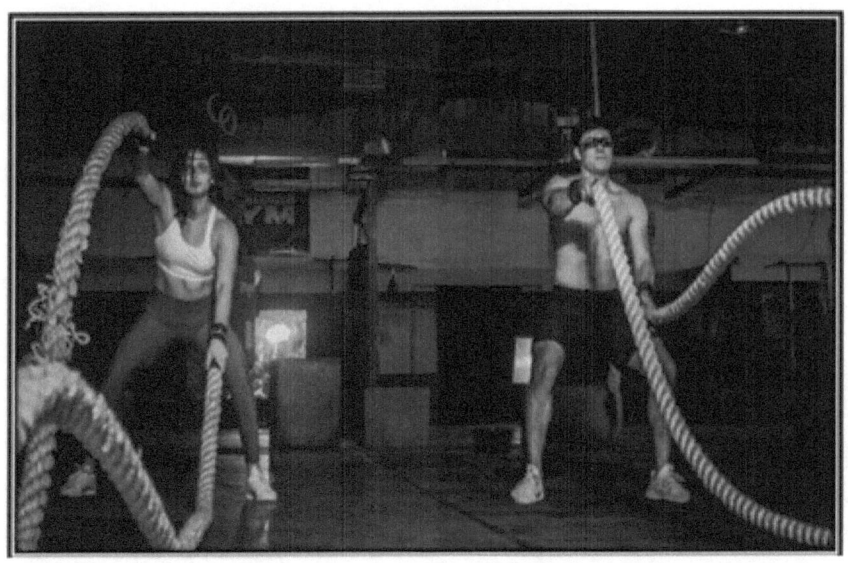

While the benefits of physical activity have long been recognized, the modern environment encourages us to pursue a lifestyle of inactivity, and poor health, evolving round altered food and air, sleep deprivation, stress and so on.

It is important to stay fit while maintaining the Paleo diet. Diet and exercise are meant to work together to bring fitness and strength. However, just like the diet, Paleo fitness is infinitely flexible and adaptable to every individual's needs.

The most important part of any exercise program is how well it works for you: Below is a list of exercises, feel free to experiment with any of the programs until you discover what best fits your abilities and goals:

Natural movement and Paleo

You should focus on your movement and not just the muscles, prioritizing activity more than exercise helps you seek health above performance.

You can achieve this by challenging yourself to a long hike, spending some quality time climbing around in a tree, or taking a swing on the monkey bars at a local playground; this allows you to have fun, amusing yourself while exercising and improving your health at the same time. Natural movement can be done anywhere, at the park, in nature of course, in your backyard, or even indoors, as long as you've learned the techniques and principles.

CrossFit and Paleo

Paleo and CrossFit are often used together. Both the paleo diet and the CrossFit exercise have their positive results, as combining both will bring amazing results within a short timeframe. CrossFit is an exercise system that involves a constant change of high-intensity workouts with routines based on movements.

Cross Fit has been the go-to regime for burning fat which involves exercises that are completed in a short time, burning more fat. You can exercise at commercial health clubs or on your own. The average exercise lasts for about two to thirty minutes.

Powerlifting and Paleo

Powerlifting involves exercises that encourage compound lifts, free weights and of course lifting heavy weights. Powerlifting also encourages utilization of natural movement to gain strength and avoid injury.

The ball is in your court; you can decide to choose any or all of these programs to aid your Paleo diet, all with a promise of improved health. Above all, rest is essential; it is important to leave plenty of time for your muscles to recover, and know when there are signs of overtraining.

Our ancestors were always on the move, and such exercises weren't around then, so understanding that movement is key will help you become as lean as your ancestors were.

CHAPTER 8

Benefits of The Paleo Diet

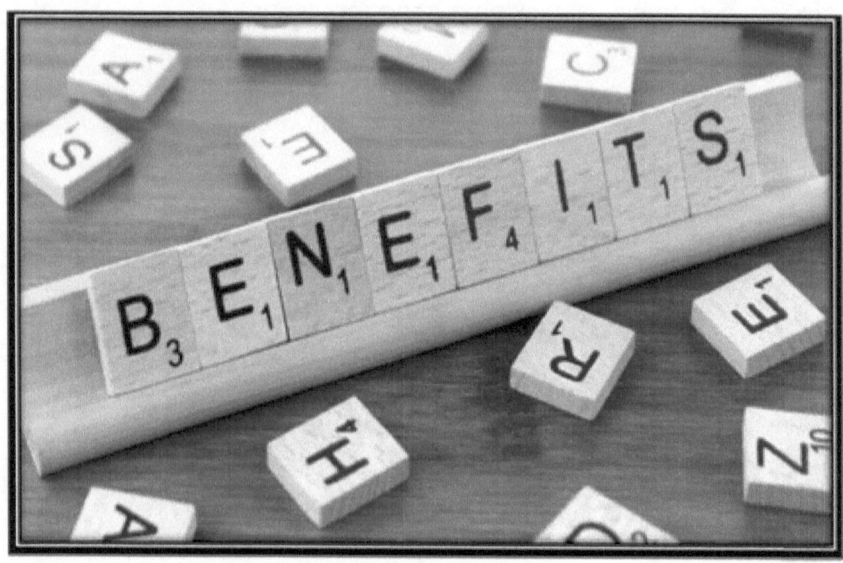

The modern diet that the human species is used to is full of preservatives, chemicals and lack nutrients that you would find in real whole foods. Eating the Paleo is about following how our ancestors ate.

They ate vegetables, grass-fed meat and while you don't notice, it now, the Paleo diet comes with a range of benefits including weight loss.

Here is how following your ancestral habits will benefit you:

Clean Eating

By eating the Paleo way, you're getting rid of processed foods and eating whole foods. The more whole foods that you eat, the more nutrients your body receives.

After a few weeks of being on the Paleo diet, you'll start to notice that you no longer crave sugar or mass quantities of carbohydrates.

Flexibility

The Paleo diet will be different for most people, but it's highly advisable that you remain active or become more active to see the benefits of what the Paleo Diet gives you.

Eating whole foods will help you take in Vitamin K, which helps calcium circulate the body. This gives you more flexibility making movement much easier.

Inflammation

The root of all evil is inflammation which is usually caused by eating processed foods. Inflammation will damage your gut which will cause your immune system to become sensitive and weak to disease.

Foods such as dairy, sugar, alcohol, and gluten cause inflammation and are eliminated because the Paleo Diet restricts those types of foods.

Cravings

If you're looking to end the cravings you have for sugary foods, the Paleo diet is a great option as more protein, and healthy fats are consumed compared to the diet of today's society.

The real whole foods that you eat stop you from experiencing blood sugar spikes and make you feel full for longer.

Sleep

The Paleo diet allows you to live a holistic lifestyle which allows you to get a good nights rest. Regular exercise and eating benefits your mind, body, and soul.

If you're struggling to sleep or suffer from insomnia, then the Paleo diet is something you need to consider.

Brain fog

Some time in your life, you'll suffer from brain fog. When this happens, you'll struggle to focus and your day becomes a disaster. There are diseases that cause brain fog, but in most cases, it's due to lack of sleep.

If you're gluten-intolerant, the Paleo diet will help by reducing brain fog as it restricts gluten completely.

Energy

After a few days of being on the Paleo diet, you'll begin to experience increased energy levels. This is due to eating natural foods full of energy and eating the right type of calories that fuel your body with the right amount of vitamins and minerals.

Foods such as eggs, nuts, and avocados contain healthy fats which help protect your brain and give it a boost.
There are many more benefits associated with the Paleo Diet including weight loss, but these were chosen to give you the motivation to get started in the quickest way possible.

CONCLUSION

You should now have an understanding of the Paleo diet, the benefits, the types of exercises that can help you get along as well as a range of foods that you need and should avoid. However, to make life easier for you, below are a few tips that will help you get started in no time.

1. Don't jump in head first. Buy a planner and slowly work your way through to become fully used to the Paleo ways.

2. Don't get rid of all your food groups in one go, this will cause your cravings to become out of control and you'll eventually give up. Instead, phase them out week by week.

3. Before you start the Paleo diet, empty all your cupboards of processed and high sugary foods.

4. Begin the diet by making one meal Paleo. For example, week 1 – only have breakfast as paleo and the rest your normal diet. Week 2 – breakfast and lunch Paleo then dinner as normal etc.

5. Make yourself a food planner and only buy the foods that you really need. A good start would be the menu at the end of Chapter 1.

6. Don't refer to the paleo diet as a diet but more of a lifestyle. Referring to it as a diet makes it sounds strict which in turn makes you nervous which you don't want to happen.

7. Invest in the right equipment, the last thing you want is not being able to prep a Paleo meal due to not having the right equipment.

8. Invest in a freezer. The Paleo diet focuses on meat so buying whole animals will become cheaper in the long run and you can ask your local butcher to chop the meat up for you.

9. Get rid of take away menu's, apps and even installing a blocker on your devices to stop you from receiving takeaway ads. The fewer distractions, the better.

10. Remember that Paleo is always meat, vegetables, and eggs. If you're eating something that falls outside these food groups, then avoid it, all together.

11. Drink plenty of water. There is enough water to go around to make sure that it's part of your diet. It's recommended you drink three liters per day.

12. Cook in batches, if you're cooking a 100% Paleo meal, prepare a lot of it. Eat what you need and freeze the rest. This helps you save time and money in the long run.

13. Although nuts do contain a high number of calories, you can get away with eating a handful three times per week.

14. Enjoy bacon and eating lots of it. Bacon contains healthy fats which is what your body needs to eat a lot of it. Take magnesium tablets if you do eat a lot of bacon.

15. Grow your herbs. Our ancestors used a lot of herbs for medical purposes but also for cooking purposes of giving their dishes a delicious taste. Consider growing your batch of parsley, thyme, basil, and rosemary on your window sill for a fresh smell every morning.

The biggest tip of all is to just simply do it. With inaction, there is no result. Make a small start today and change each day as you go. Soon you'll be wearing a caveman outfit enjoying the range of benefits that come with it.

Good Luck!

Now You are on You're Way To A Paleo Lifestyle!

Thank You For Reading